CW00970723

NICOLE RONSARD'S No-Excuse Exercise Guide

WILLIAM MORROW AND COMPANY, INC. • NEW YORK

By the same author—
CELLULITE: THOSE LUMPS,
BUMPS AND BULGES
YOU COULDN'T LOSE BEFORE

Credits:
Edited by Mary Butler
Illustrations: Anna Marie Magagna
Cover and book design: Kennetha Stewart
Hand lettering: Jean Hipp

Printed in the United States of America.

1 2 3 4 5 80 79 78 77 76

Library of Congress Catalog Card Number 75–33480

ISBN 0–688–03020–3

CONTENTS

FOREWORD

Today's world banishes taboos, glorifies the body. Good. Today, a woman can be proud of her body instead of, as in the past, having to ignore, hide, compress and corset it. But a proud body requires some care.

In my first book, *Cellulite: Those Lumps, Bumps and Bulges You Couldn't Lose Before,* I outlined a complete six-point program—proper diet, increase of elimination, correct breathing, exercise geared to the trouble spots, massage and relaxation—to control and eliminate this common figure problem. Cellulite is prevalent today because we don't use our bodies. We eat "junk foods," processed foods that do more harm than good for the figure . . . then sit around—in cars, behind desks, in front of TV's. No wonder the body rebels. But cellulite is not the only result of bad "body" habits. A figure can be cellulite-free and still be out of shape.

This book is for day-in and day-out body shaping. It is not a cellulite control regime by any means. The inspiration came about as a direct result of the figure problem discussions I had with thousands and thousands of women throughout America. I felt there ought to be a simple, easy way to keep in shape. While all too many women want to "do something" about their figures, I've heard over and over comments like "I really don't have time to exercise," "I have a family that keeps me busy enough," "I'm too tired after work to make time to exercise," and "I know I should but I just don't get around to it."

Here's the answer. A fresh approach designed to fit right into the way women live, work and play in today's world. It's simple, it's easy to follow. The idea is to try to make use of any moment of the day to give your muscles quick, effective workouts. Wherever you are: in the office, your kitchen, your car. While doing something else: talking on the phone, typing, reading, doing housework or soaking in the tub. Even lying down watching TV.

I wanted to capture this fresh new approach in the pages of a book, but not an ordinary exercise book. So you'll see pictures that integrate exercise into all aspects of daily life, that make exercise look as inviting as it really is. Not the boring routine it usually is.

I call it the *No-Excuse Exercise Guide.* I hope it will convince you that exercise can be fun. That you can stay in shape without much fuss or bother, here, there and everywhere. So take stock now…no more of that "no time" routine. You really have No Excuse to be out of shape!

THE GAME PLAN

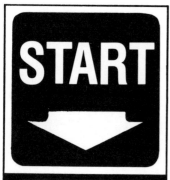

START

LOVE YOURSELF

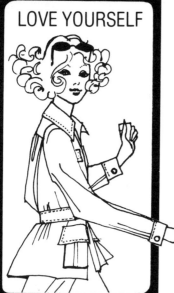

because you are you...
you are unique,
a very special, very
precious person.

then

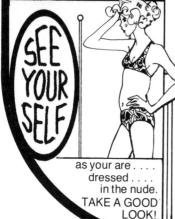

SEE YOUR SELF

as your are . . . .
dressed . . . .
in the nude.
TAKE A GOOD
LOOK!

**now...
DO YOU RATE?**

Find out where you could
trim a little, add a little . . . .
IMPROVE A LOT!

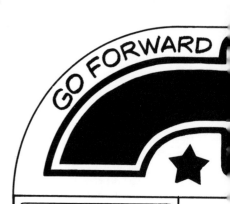

GO FORWARD

FOR COMFORT

1.

Clothes that FIT right
make you FEEL right.
Choose the right type of
clothes for <u>your</u> figure,
<u>your</u> way of living.

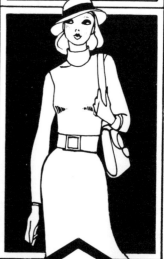

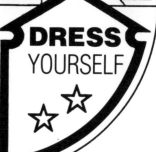

DRESS YOURSELF

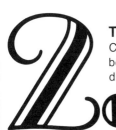

2. **TO FLATTER**
Clothes should enhance your body. Naturally. <u>NOT</u> disguise or camouflage it!

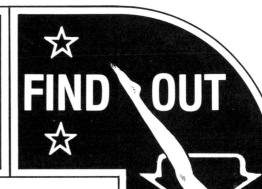

FIND OUT

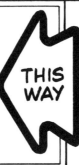

It's HOW, <u>not</u> how many, that makes EXERCISE work!

THIS WAY

What's NEW about EXERCISE!

ADD IT ALL UP!

You get the shape you want and more…

1. body control
2. a feeling of pleasure
3. a feeling of satisfaction
4. more self-confidence

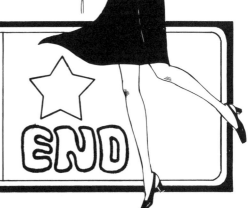

MEET THE BEAUTIFUL YOU!

Every woman CAN be beautiful. All you need is the will to make it happen. As for the know-how . . . now there's NO-EXCUSE!

END

7

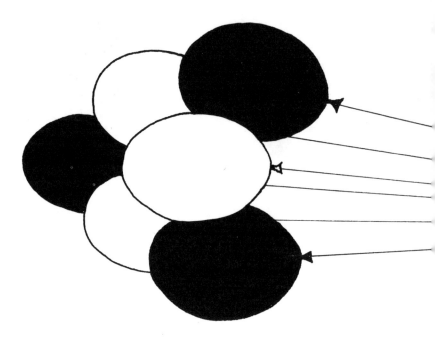

LOVE YOURSELF

Your body is your most precious possession. Priceless. Be kind to it. Give it all the care and attention it needs. With pleasure.

Love your body. There's nothing wrong with that. On the contrary. You must love yourself before others can love you. You must feel good about yourself. Happy with what you have. What you see. This is not being narcissistic. It's being just plain normal.

This is what we French call "être bien dans sa peau" (to feel good in one's skin). When you feel good about yourself, you are sure of yourself. Cool. Poised. You move gracefully, carry your body lightly. Sensuously. As it was meant to be.

This, in turn, will reflect in everything you do. Your personality will be different. More pleasant. This is really what is meant by being attractive. It's what emanates from you that makes you beautiful.

Love yourself. Everybody will love you more for it.

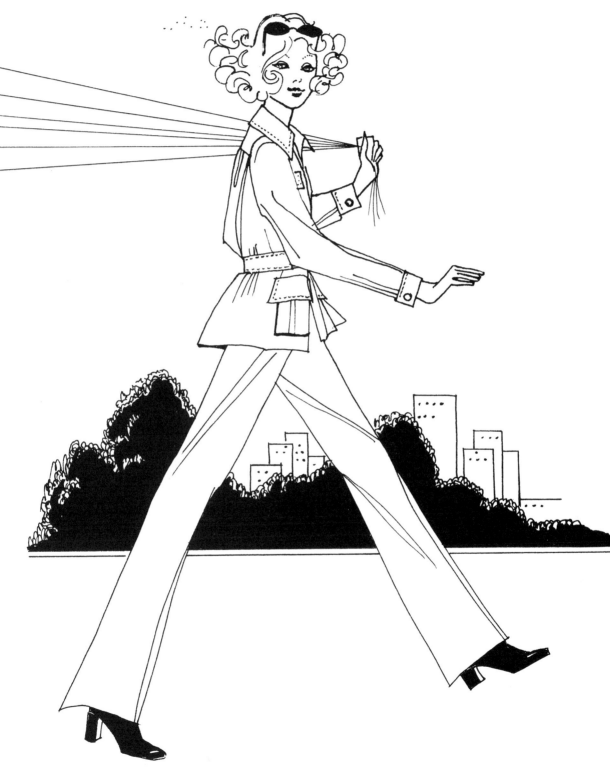

MIRROR, MIRROR...

A skinny body is not necessarily a beautiful body. You were born with a certain bone structure . . . which you cannot change. Whether or not it fits your beauty criteria. We have been brainwashed into thinking we should all look like fashion models. Skin and bones.

This is so far from reality.

You are *you*. You are unique.

Make the most of what you were born with. That's what it's all about. Once you've decided you're worth the work, taking care of yourself becomes an integral part of your daily routine. Every woman CAN be beautiful. All you need is the will to do it. And with the know-how, you can actually "sculpt" your body.

HOW DO YOU RATE?

(CHECK)

□ Thighs—smooth and shapely?   □ Thighs—flabby?
□ Buttocks—trim?   □ Buttocks—falling?
□ Stomach—flat?   □ Stomach—protruding?
□ Back—straight?   □ Back—hunched?
□ Bust—uplifted?   □ Bust—droopy?
□ Upper arms—taut?   □ Upper arms—shapeless?
□ Shoulders—back?   □ Shoulders—slumped?
□ Chin—firm?   □ Chin—sagging, double?
□ "Swan" neck?   □ Crepey neck?
□ Head—erect?   □ Head—bent?

You should not think of yourself in terms of being dressed all the time. Because you're not. You should look and feel as beautiful in the nude as you do when you're dressed. Even more so.

You look at your face in the mirror at least every morning and evening. You know exactly what you look like, made-up and "au naturel." How often do you look at your body? Naked? Take a close look. And not only from the front. From the back too. Be aware of your body.

THE MOMENT OF TRUTH...the fitting room.

The best time to take stock . . . when you're trying on clothes, underwear or a bathing suit especially. You're surrounded by mirrors. The lighting is awful. You look awful. You feel terrible. There's no place to hide. You wonder if this is really you. What happened to the beautiful, slim, shapely girl you once knew? Excuses. Excuses. Excuses. Now's the time. There's NO EXCUSE.

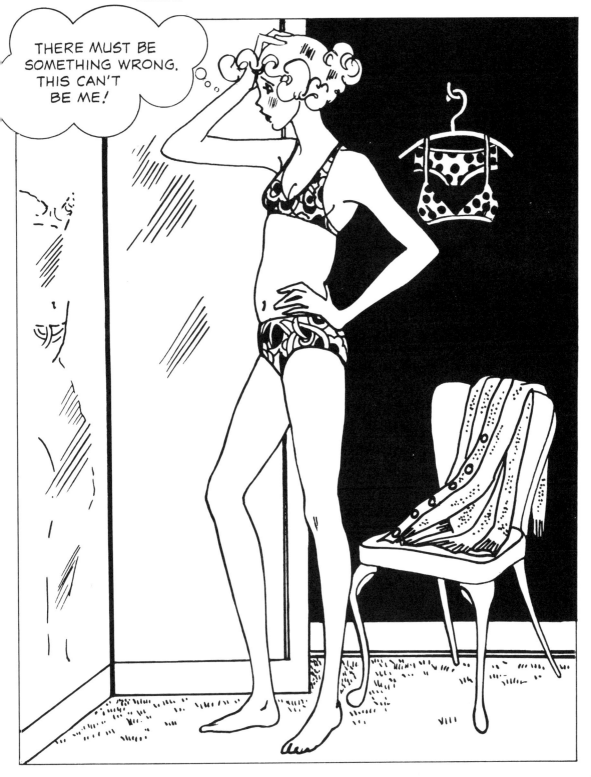

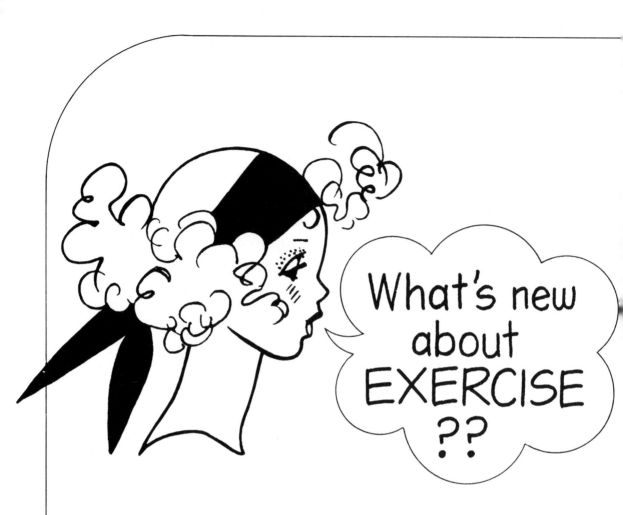

What's new about EXERCISE ??

A lot. The attitude toward exercise for one thing. Exercise is "in." Almost everyone is doing something active. You can stand up, sit down, lie down, all in the name of exercise. You don't have to follow boring "1-2-3, 1-2-3," military type routines, sweating and straining, ending up exhausted to get results.

EXERCISE "builds" muscles, of course. Women don't like to hear that. But the effect on the feminine figure is splendid—it firms, shapes, uplifts. Though men and women share the same muscle system, a woman has an extra layer of fat that keeps her smooth and rounded. Thoroughly female.

EXERCISE has come out of the closet and into daily life. No longer does it need special settings, special clothes, special times. Exercise is only as special as you make it.

EXERCISE is movement. Movement is exercise *if you make it so.* As you move through your day, at home, at work or at play, you can exercise simply, quickly and easily. Think of exercise as the prevention that beats the cure.

EXERCISE need no longer be tedious or boring to give results. You must know the right movements, and do them faithfully and regularly. There actually comes a time when exercise becomes pleasant to do. It's a great feeling. A feeling of being closer to your body. More aware.

Just think of the countless, precious minutes you could make good use of . . . instead of just "wishing you had the time to exercise."

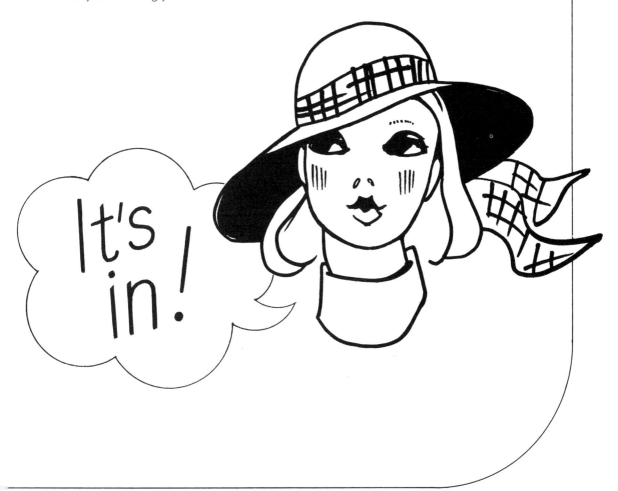

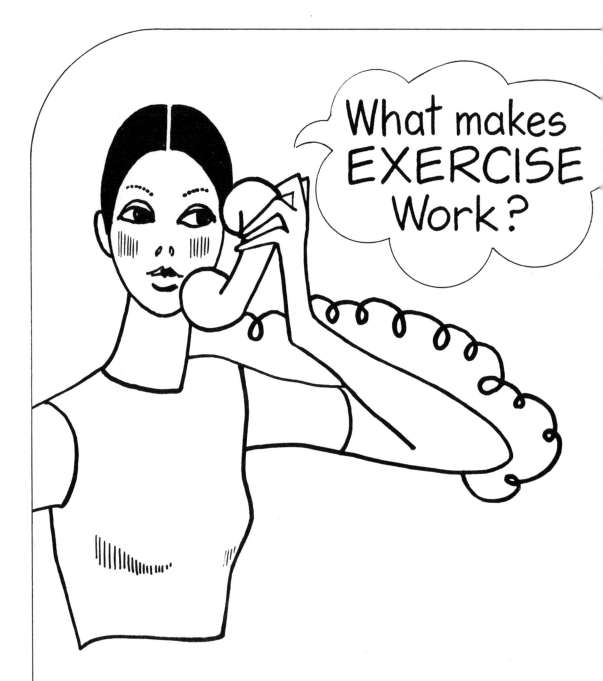

Your enthusiasm. Getting started is hardly the problem. It's sticking to your resolution that's the hard part. For exercise to be beneficial, you needn't spend an hour a day, nor do you have to suffer through countless movements. But you do need the right ones. And you do need to do them regularly, ideally every day.

Your concentration. It is actually concentration that makes the difference in whether a movement gives results or not. Do every movement fully. Feel your muscles stretch and contract. Feel them pulling and exaggerate the movement voluntarily. This makes it twice as effective.

Your persistence. Start. Stop. Start again . . . This gets you nowhere. And your poor body gets its signals crossed. Spending even a few minutes a day, but every day, regularly, is bound to show results.

Your common sense. Be sensible. You will not be able to repair years of neglect in just a few days. But if you really put your mind to it and stick to your program, it will work. And here's where the NO-EXCUSE Plan comes to your aid. It fits right into the way you live, the way you work and play.

And one more thing about getting results: you must do every movement the best you can. And you must believe in what you're doing.

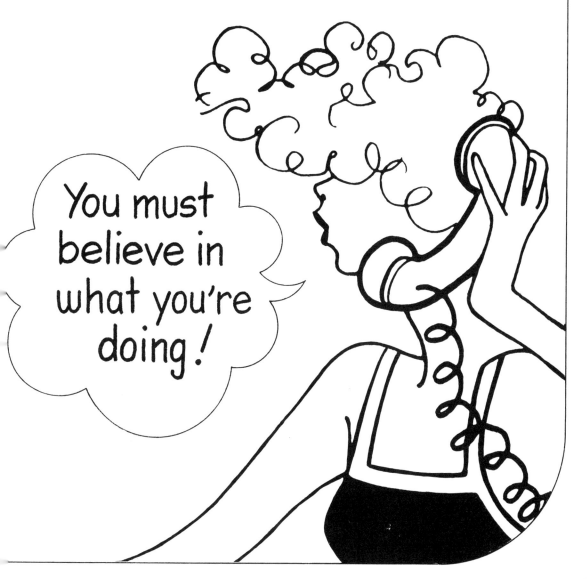

You must believe in what you're doing!

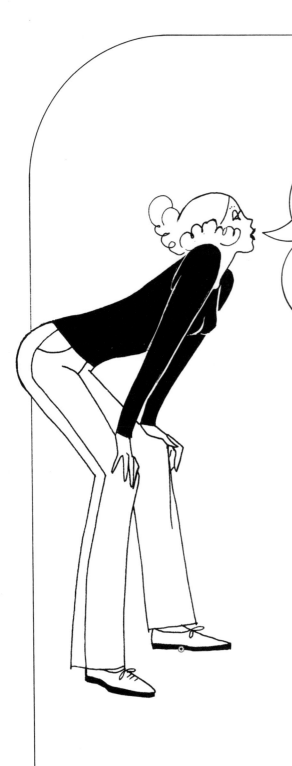

What you get out of exercise.

- a firm, shapely figure
- good, healthy circulation
- deep, natural sleep
- easy, supple movement
- lithe, youthful posture
- tensions are reduced
- energy is increased
- muscle tone improves
- sensual awareness expands
- you feel all-over alive PHYSICALLY!

And Puritanism aside, your body does function better all around when you use it. It wa designed to be used, to walk, to talk, to think, to eat, sleep and make love. And almost everythir the body does requires movement. All that movement is exercise if you want it to be. You g out of it what you put into it. No more. No less.

- you feel a new sense of body pleasure
- you have more confidence
- you find a positive self awareness
- your outlook on living improves
- your satisfaction with self increases
- you find it's easier to think clearly
- you find it easier to act
- reactions are more positive than negative
- feelings of real accomplishment happen more often
- when body and mind are one, you're all together PSYCHOLOGICALLY!

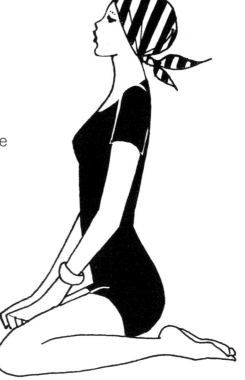

Thanks to Dr. Freud, we all know how big a part the mind plays on the body and vice versa. One cannot exist without the other. If you work on your body you're going to work on your mind whether you plan to or not. So concentrate on the positive feeling that you are worth doing something special for. And the results will make it all worthwhile.

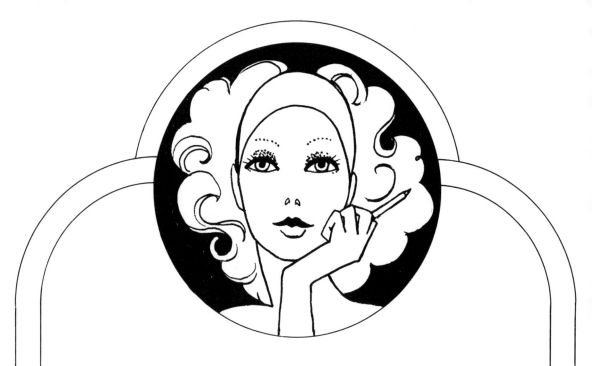

MY TIPS FOR SUCCESS

SET A GOAL

You want your body to look better. Firmer. Shapelier. You must work at it. It's not all that difficult. But you must motivate yourself.

At Home
Work in front of a mirror. This helps you make sure that you're doing the movements properly. Especially at first. It also makes exercise more interesting. Watch closely how you move. Study yourself. Make your movements graceful. Fluid. Not drill type.

In the Nude
If you like, work out in the nude. It's a very sensuous experience.

Feeling Lazy?
When your will power is getting low, talk to yourself. Tell yourself, "You're lazy, you're just looking for an excuse to skip your exercises." Remind yourself, "If you don't do this yourself, nobody is going to do it for you."

Don't Look
You'll only be discouraged if you keep looking in the mirror every day to see improvement. Give it a little time.

Don't Despair
Remember, a new figure doesn't happen overnight. Keep up the good work.

YOU'LL IMPROVE—FOR SURE!

DISCOVER
A
NEW
YOU...
INSTANTLY!

None of us would think of driving a car or using a precision tool if the parts were not in their proper place. And yet this is exactly what we do to our bodies every day of our lives.

Posture can help you discover a new you *instantly*. Posture is a major key to beauty. It is *the* secret and yet very few of us take full advantage of it. It is the most powerful beauty and health tool we own. What a terrible mistake to misuse or not use it. Either from ignorance or neglect. How sad.

In the minds of most of us, good posture implies "army" type, ramrod stiffness. In reality, it means grace, poise, suppleness, proud carriage of the body—whether you stand, walk, sit or bend. Good posture is just proper alignment of the body. The way it is meant to be. The best way to learn proper posture is to practice in front of a mirror, in profile. And what should you look like if you have good posture?

Spine stretched,
chest up,
shoulders back but relaxed,
neck stretched,
head comfortably centered over the spine,
buttocks tucked in slightly,
stomach pulled in and up, nice and flat,
knees slightly bent,
weight of the body resting on the balls of the feet.

This might feel awkward at first. And to get it right will require concentration. Bad lifelong postural habits cannot be changed overnight. But once you get the feel of it, this will become instinctive.

The way your body ultimately shapes up depends a lot on good posture or proper use of your body. Just think of the innumerable times you have to sit down, stand up or bend your body during a day. Make good use of those movements instead of just throwing, flopping or dragging yourself around. Transform them into "exercises"—which is exactly what they're supposed to be. Make the most of them.

"Think" each one of your movements instead of going around like a robot. And always remember to stand, walk and sit "tall." This allows all the parts of your body—organs, bones, nerves, blood vessels, muscles—to assume their proper place and perform their various tasks correctly. It gives you more energy and vitality and a better outlook on life in general.

To sum it up, good posture gives your body an "instant lift." A total "remake."

GOOD POSTURE CAN:

- Make you look younger, thinner, more attractive, graceful, poised, relaxed.

- Free you from tension and save you many aches and pains.

- Reduce fatigue and strain.

- Tone and firm muscles.

- Smooth out a neckline.

- Lift your breasts and buttocks.

- Flatten your stomach.

- Afford better digestion and elimination.

- Improve circulation.

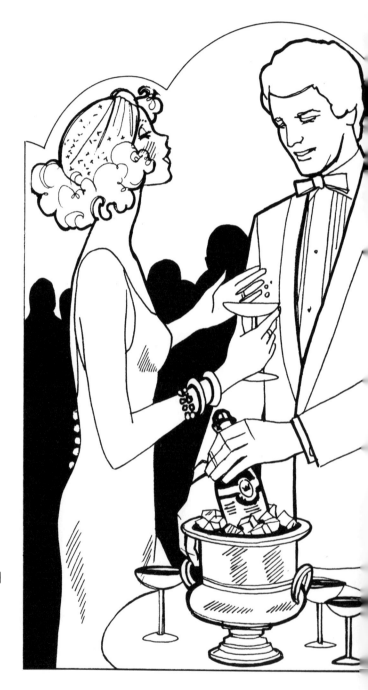

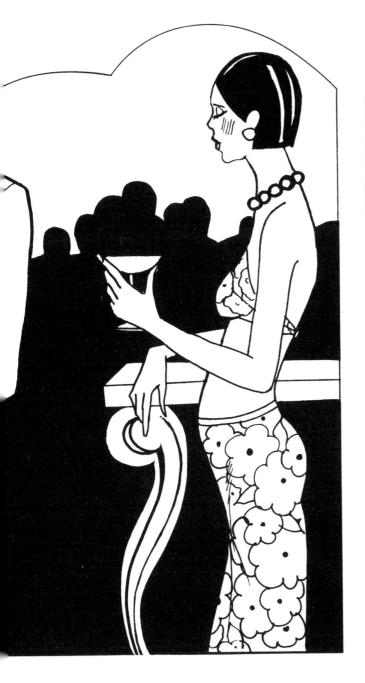

BAD POSTURE DOES:

- Make you look dumpy, awkward, defeated, strained, ill-at-ease.

- Increase tension and create unnecessary aches, pains and muscle fatigue.

- Make for poor muscle tone.

- Create a double chin.

- Cause a dowager's hump.

- Make breasts and buttocks sag.

- Result in a protruding abdomen, and/or a sway back, back pains.

- Interfere with proper digestion and elimination.

- Impede good circulation.

SITTING

The very action of sitting and standing, when done properly, actually exercises and firms muscles, shapes and molds the body. When you sit, do it right: back erect and supported by the back of the chair. Stomach pulled in. Weight of the body resting on the sitz bones. To find the exact point for comfortable sitting, fidget on the seat of your chair until you feel the two bones located at the bottom of the buttocks.

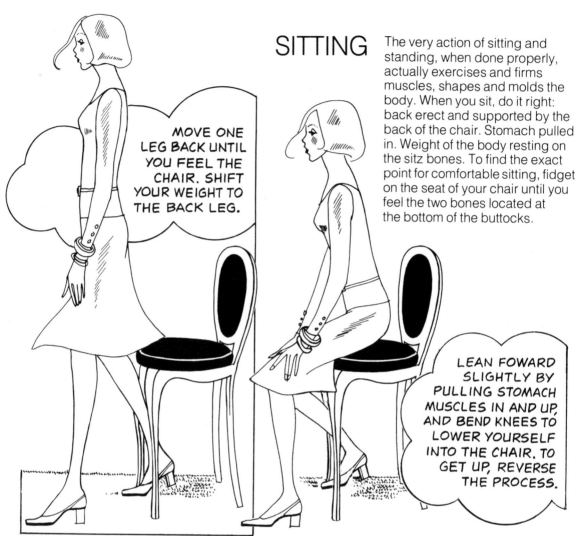

MOVE ONE LEG BACK UNTIL YOU FEEL THE CHAIR. SHIFT YOUR WEIGHT TO THE BACK LEG.

LEAN FOWARD SLIGHTLY BY PULLING STOMACH MUSCLES IN AND UP, AND BEND KNEES TO LOWER YOURSELF INTO THE CHAIR. TO GET UP, REVERSE THE PROCESS.

SITTING BADLY IS TERRIBLY DESTRUCTIVE TO THE BODY. FIGURE-WISE *AND* HEALTH-WISE.

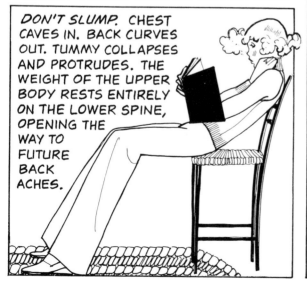

DON'T SLUMP. CHEST CAVES IN. BACK CURVES OUT. TUMMY COLLAPSES AND PROTRUDES. THE WEIGHT OF THE UPPER BODY RESTS ENTIRELY ON THE LOWER SPINE, OPENING THE WAY TO FUTURE BACK ACHES.

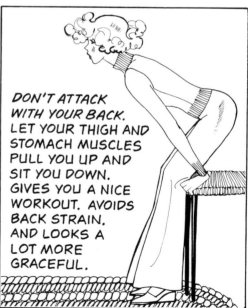

DON'T ATTACK WITH YOUR BACK. LET YOUR THIGH AND STOMACH MUSCLES PULL YOU UP AND SIT YOU DOWN. GIVES YOU A NICE WORKOUT. AVOIDS BACK STRAIN. AND LOOKS A LOT MORE GRACEFUL.

WALKING

You get as much out of walking as you put into it. It becomes a super exercise when you concentrate on walking with your whole body. And the secret is to swing your leg from the hip—not the knee—in one smooth motion. Keep your stomach pulled in and your back straight, shoulders and arms relaxed.

Walking like this in comfortable shoes (not two-story-high fashion clogs) is exhilarating. The perfect body pick-up.

For extra benefits: tense your inner thighs and buttocks with each step.

BENDING FOR BEAUTY

Always bend knees slightly when leaning over. Pull stomach in as your body goes forward. Put one foot in front of the other for balance. Use thigh and buttock muscles to lower and raise yourself. Exercise like that really helps.

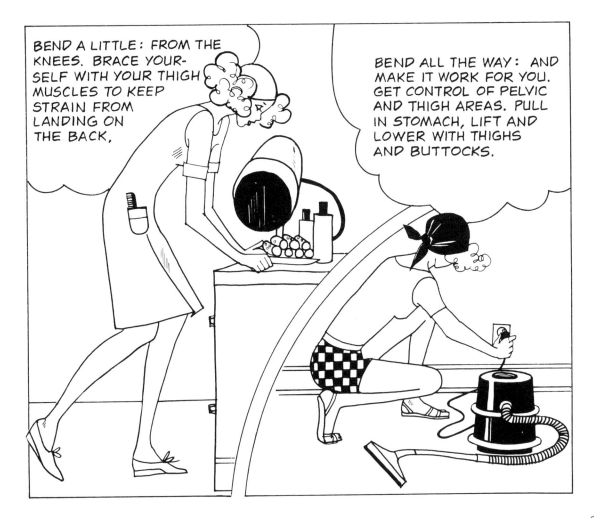

DAILY LIFE is full of "no-nos."

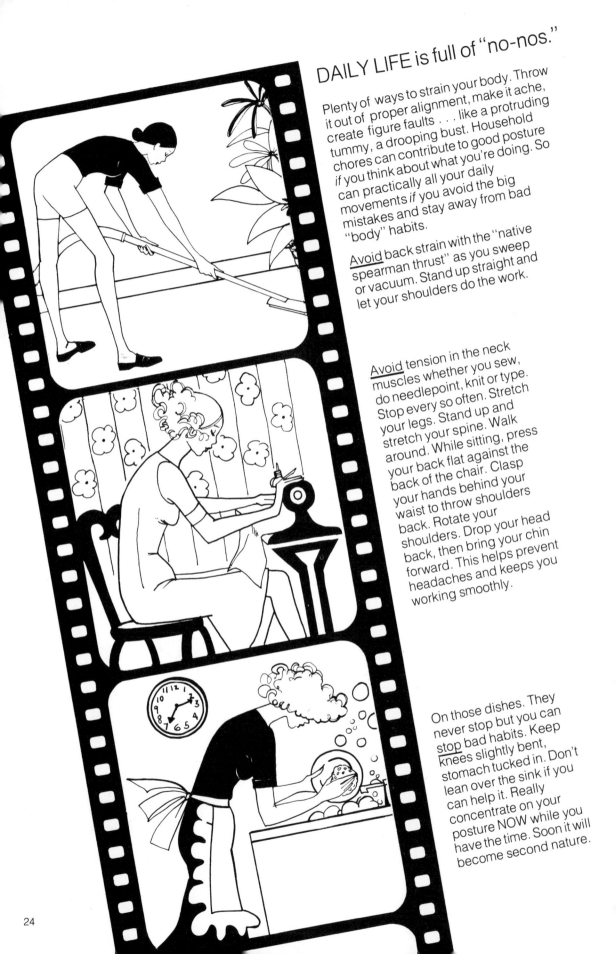

Plenty of ways to strain your body. Throw it out of proper alignment, make it ache, create figure faults . . . like a protruding tummy, a drooping bust. Household chores can contribute to good posture if you think about what you're doing. So can practically all your daily movements if you avoid the big mistakes and stay away from bad "body" habits.

Avoid back strain with the "native spearman thrust" as you sweep or vacuum. Stand up straight and let your shoulders do the work.

Avoid tension in the neck muscles whether you sew, do needlepoint, knit or type. Stop every so often. Stretch your legs. Stand up and stretch your spine. Walk around. While sitting, press your back flat against the back of the chair. Clasp your hands behind your waist to throw shoulders back. Rotate your shoulders. Drop your head back, then bring your chin forward. This helps prevent headaches and keeps you working smoothly.

On those dishes. They never stop but you can stop bad habits. Keep knees slightly bent, stomach tucked in. Don't lean over the sink if you can help it. Really concentrate on your posture NOW while you have the time. Soon it will become second nature.

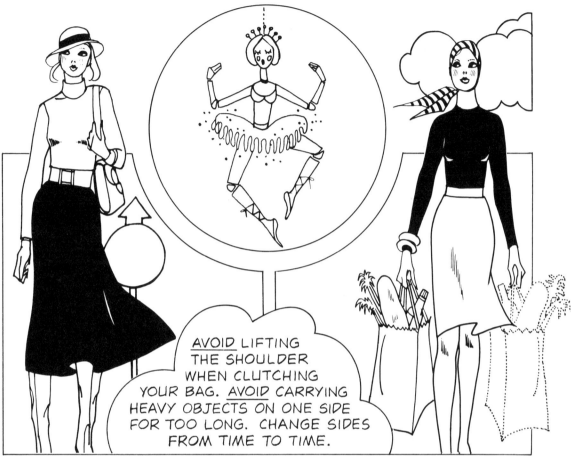

AVOID LIFTING THE SHOULDER WHEN CLUTCHING YOUR BAG. AVOID CARRYING HEAVY OBJECTS ON ONE SIDE FOR TOO LONG. CHANGE SIDES FROM TIME TO TIME.

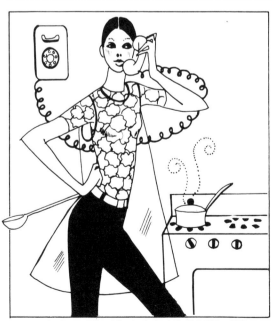

AVOID STANDING ON ONE FOOT. IT THROWS YOUR BODY OUT OF KILTER.

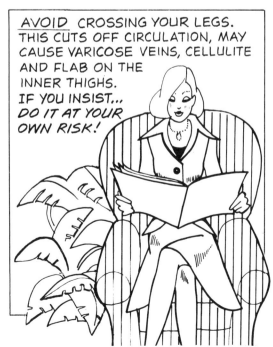

AVOID CROSSING YOUR LEGS. THIS CUTS OFF CIRCULATION, MAY CAUSE VARICOSE VEINS, CELLULITE AND FLAB ON THE INNER THIGHS. IF YOU INSIST... DO IT AT YOUR OWN RISK!

25

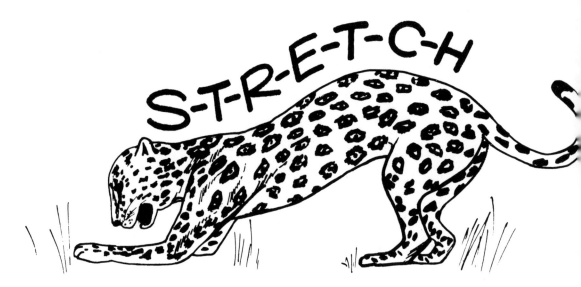

...THAT NEW YOU INTO SHAPE

You've looked. And you've learned how to "remake" your body through good posture. Now let's keep it on the right track by stretching.

STRETCHING is the most natural form of movement. Just look at a cat stretching from tip to tail. Try to copy some of its movements. You'll feel a release all over.

STRETCHING is instinctive in children too and it's a pity we lose that vital instinct as we grow older and more "disciplined."

STRETCHING is the surest way to keep young and supple. The safest way to ward off aching/tight muscles, tension, fatigue, even injury from sudden movements:

INTEGRATE STRETCHING INTO YOUR DAILY MOVEMENTS:

- Making a bed
- Lifting a child
- Filing office reports
- Going through a doorway
- Reaching for something
- On the phone
- In the tub
- In the car
- At the movies
- In front of the TV

STRETCHING makes you feel tall, lissome, slinky, relaxed . . . and definitely sexy.

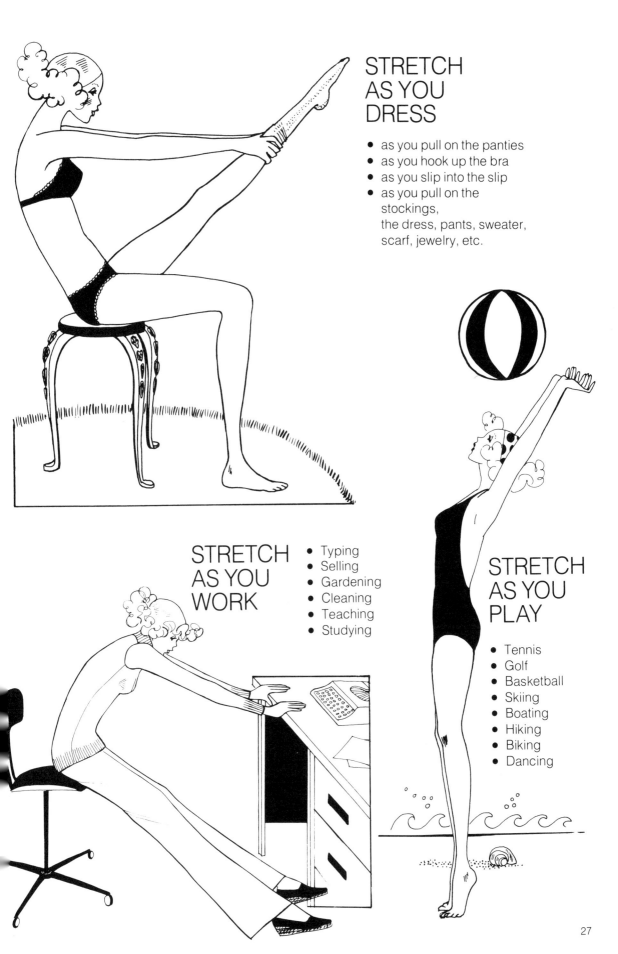

STRETCH AS YOU DRESS

- as you pull on the panties
- as you hook up the bra
- as you slip into the slip
- as you pull on the stockings,
  the dress, pants, sweater,
  scarf, jewelry, etc.

STRETCH AS YOU WORK

- Typing
- Selling
- Gardening
- Cleaning
- Teaching
- Studying

STRETCH AS YOU PLAY

- Tennis
- Golf
- Basketball
- Skiing
- Boating
- Hiking
- Biking
- Dancing

27

BRUSH AND STRETCH

BRUSH YOUR HAIR, BENDING FROM THE WAIST TO RELEASE LOWER BACK TENSION. BOUNCE GENTLY AND BRING NATURE'S OWN BLUSH TO YOUR FACE.

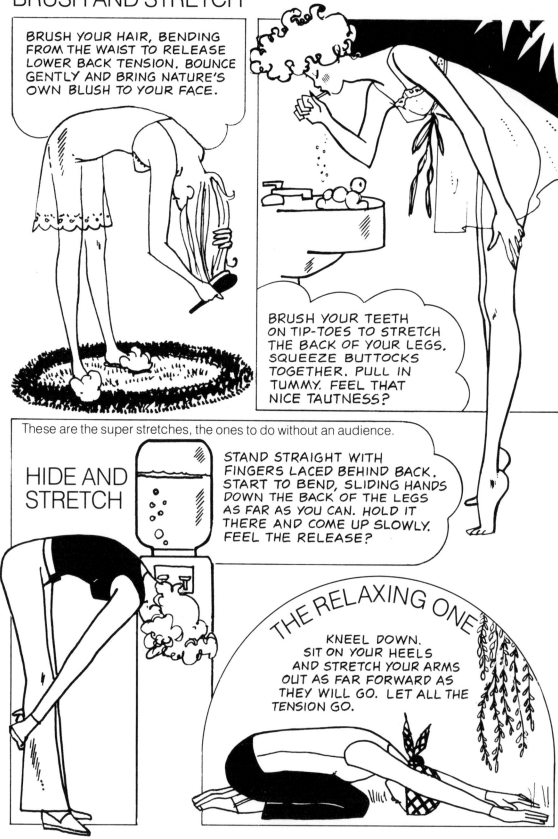

BRUSH YOUR TEETH ON TIP-TOES TO STRETCH THE BACK OF YOUR LEGS. SQUEEZE BUTTOCKS TOGETHER. PULL IN TUMMY. FEEL THAT NICE TAUTNESS?

These are the super stretches, the ones to do without an audience.

HIDE AND STRETCH

STAND STRAIGHT WITH FINGERS LACED BEHIND BACK. START TO BEND, SLIDING HANDS DOWN THE BACK OF THE LEGS AS FAR AS YOU CAN. HOLD IT THERE AND COME UP SLOWLY. FEEL THE RELEASE?

THE RELAXING ONE

KNEEL DOWN. SIT ON YOUR HEELS AND STRETCH YOUR ARMS OUT AS FAR FORWARD AS THEY WILL GO. LET ALL THE TENSION GO.

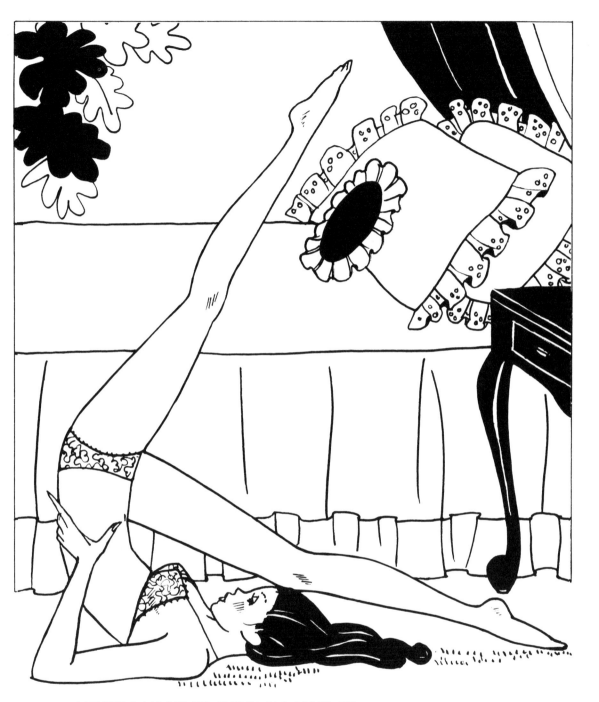

WHEN YOU'VE REALLY HAD IT...

HERE'S SOMETHING TO PICK YOU UP. GO INTO YOUR BEDROOM, BATHROOM, OFFICE... CLOSE THE DOOR AND LIE DOWN ON YOUR BACK. SWING YOUR HIPS OFF THE FLOOR AND SLOWLY MOVE YOUR LEGS BACK AND FORTH, SIDE BY SIDE, FLEX YOUR KNEES, DO A SPLIT. BRACE YOUR HIPS WITH YOUR HANDS. THIS REVERSES THE PULL OF GRAVITY. AND GIVES YOU A WHOLE NEW OUTLOOK ON THINGS. *BEATS A FIVE O'CLOCK MARTINI!*

THINK STRETCHING

...as you walk:

- ☐ Go around the house on tip-toe.
- ☐ Keep knees stiff, stay on tip-toe. Keep stomach in, buttocks tucked under.
- ☐ Walk like a pigeon, tip-toes IN, knees stiff (feel the inner thigh tighten).
- ☐ Reverse. Go like a duck, tip-toes OUT, knees stiff (feel that stretch on the outer thigh).

...as you climb:

Use those stairs to trim your legs and stretch away tension.

- ☐ Go *up* stairs, lifting as you go. On each step, place foot securely, then rise on toes.
- ☐ Criss-cross legs, one over the other, still rising up on your toes, one step at a time. Or keep feet flat (feel the pull on both inside *and* outside thigh).
- ☐ Go *down* stairs, standing "tall," not hunched over like an old lady. Land on your toes *or* on your heels all the way down.
    What a way to stretch out the legs!

...as you do your thing:

Improvise. Innovate. Stretch . . . Stretch . . . Stretch . . .
You feel better. You look better.

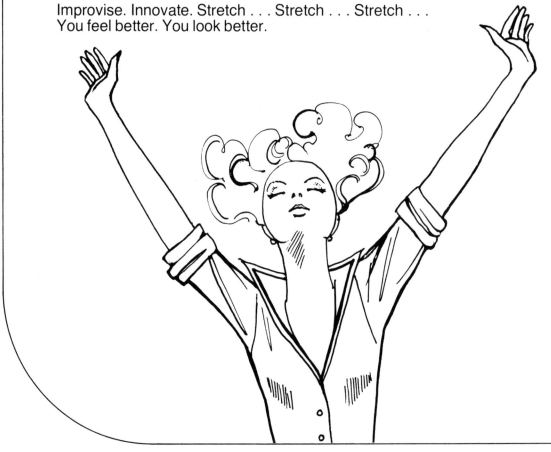

AREA CODES

And now, to the specifics. Up to now, we've talked about the whole body. Helping to put it in shape, make it look good all over. That's important. But if you have problem areas, you want to get right to work on them, make them look as good as possible as quickly as possible.

Each area has its own special requirements—its own special movements. You can do most of them easily, as part of your daily routine. They adapt to your way of living and moving as they work to solve your problems. Some exercises require privacy and concentration. But they are included because they speed up results.

HERE'S HOW I RATE THE DIFFERENT AREAS:

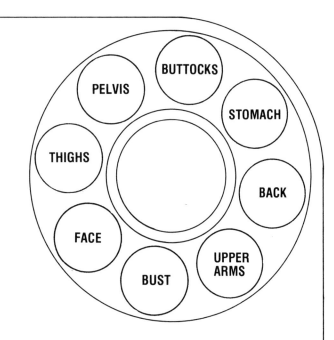

THIGHS   If they're cellulite-free—you see firmer, shapelier thighs with remarkable speed.

PELVIS   Slower—but not unbeatable.

UTTOCKS   Difficult—so persevere.

STOMACH   You can see this one so you concentrate harder. And here posture—good posture—cuts the job by half.

BACK   Posture helps here too. And exercise keeps the back supple, tension-free, prevents flab from collecting around the hips, by the bra.

UPPER ARMS   The sooner you get started on these, the better. Tricky, once they deteriorate.

BUST   You cannot increase . . . or decrease your size but you *can* stay firm. Exercise gives you the support you need for a young-looking bustline.

FACE   Start now. Don't let lines, tension, sagging get a head start. You *can* slow down premature aging . . . if you care enough!

YOU AND YOUR THIGHS

A big problem, if you're cellulite-prone. Then you need more than simple exercise. You should follow the six-point, cellulite-correction plan outlined in my book *Cellulite: Those Lumps, Bumps and Bulges You Couldn't Lose Before.*

But in many cases, thighs are just plain flabby. Especially when you lose weight. They need to be firmed up. Toned. Trimmed. These exercises will do the job. And you can do them quickly, easily, anywhere, just about any time of day.

With a minimum of effort you exercise the whole thigh as you sit, walk, bend, play sports. But the inner thigh, *that's something else.* Here are a few everyday hints:

SITTING DOWN—thighs together, feet about 10 inches apart, toes turned out, press knees together as hard as you can. Hold. Slowly release. Repeat.

STANDING—feet about 4 inches apart, knees slightly bent, toes turned in, try to bring legs together without moving feet. Remember though, there is no movement involved.

FOLLOW THE NO-EXCUSE METHOD* FOR MAXIMUM RESULTS:

1. Go S-L-O-W-L-Y. This is crucial.
2. When movements call for **HOLD**, start counting by hundreds—101-102-103. Slowly. Build holding time up to 110/120.
3. **REPEAT** each movement 3 to 5 times to start. As you improve, aim for at least 10 times.

*The NO-EXCUSE METHOD applies to all the exercises in this book.

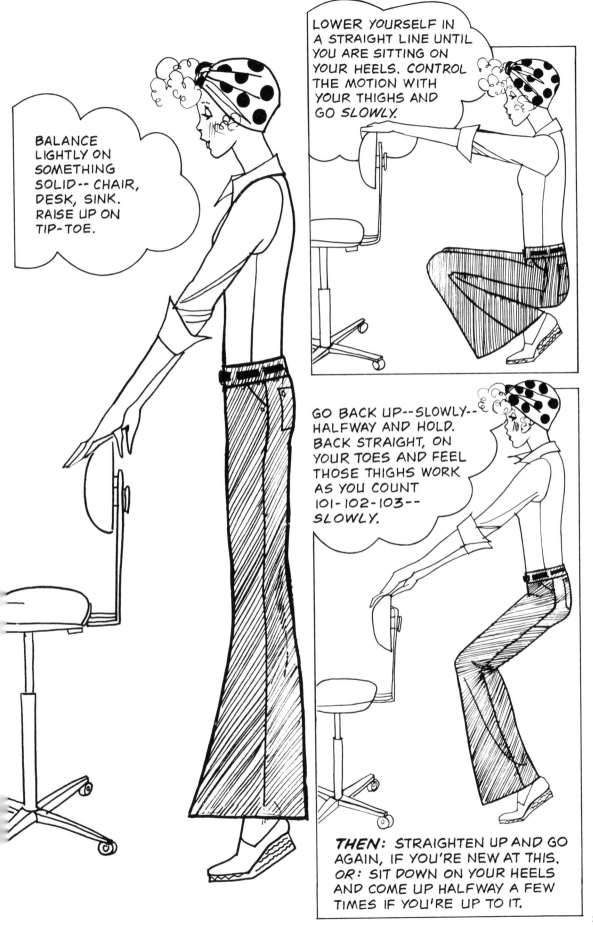

THIGH SAVERS

SITTING. STRAIGHT, OF COURSE. RAISE ONE LEG TO HIP LEVEL. HOLD IT THERE KEEPING KNEE STIFF. SLOWLY COUNT TO 5. WORK UP TO 20. VARIATIONS: LEG IN SAME POSITION-- 1. MAKE TINY BOUNCE MOVEMENTS⬍. 2. CIRCLE FEET FROM ANKLES. 3. FLEX FEET.

BALLERINAS USE THESE TRICKS TO KEEP LEGS FIRM AND STRONG. YOU CAN TOO-- WHILE READING, WATCHING TV, ON THE PHONE!

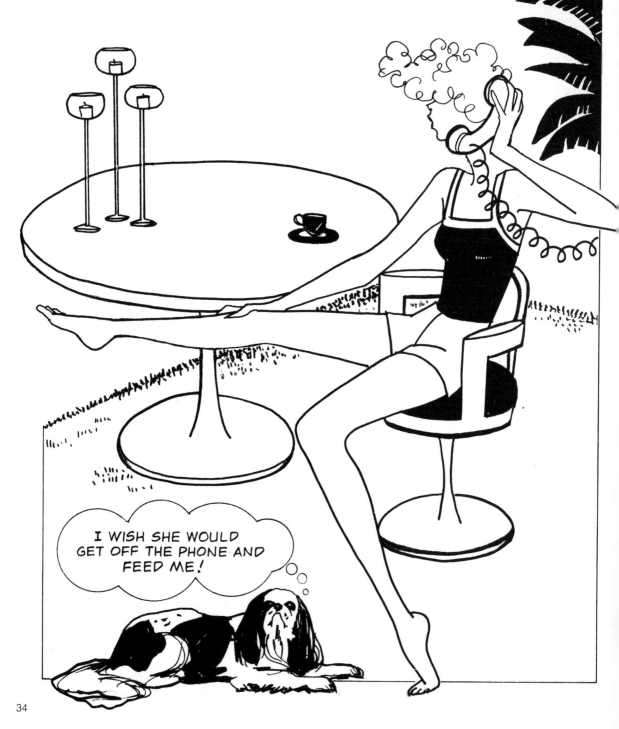

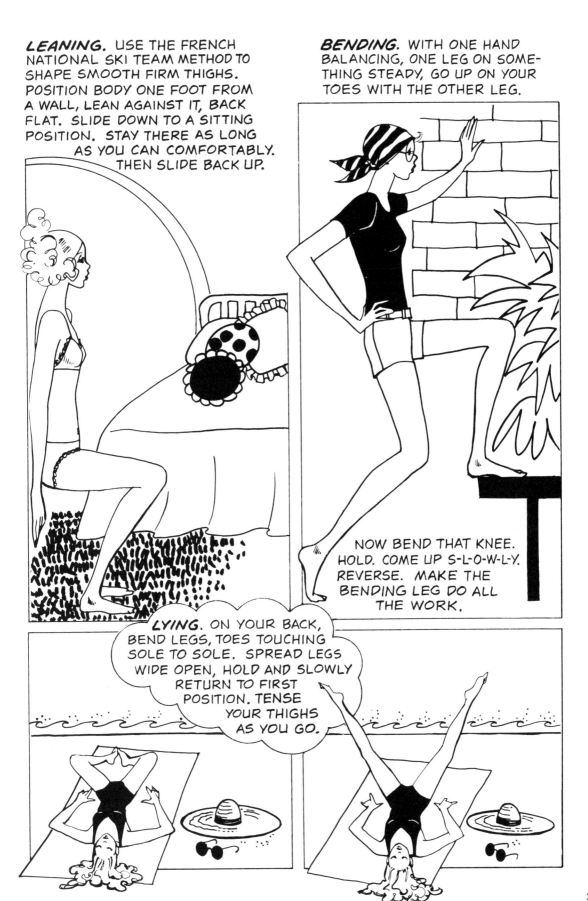

FIRST AID FOR INNER THIGHS

The inner thigh is one of the most delicate areas of a woman's body . . . one that deteriorates rapidly, even at an early age, if not given constant attention.

Yet very few exercises and practically no sports bring this area into play. Even more disturbing, inner thighs get no exercise at all in day-to-day living . . . a flabby, out-of-shape, chronic trouble spot for practically everyone.

After extensive research and testing, I developed MultiToner * to do what ordinary exercise can't do. MultiToner works directly on those hard-to-reach problem areas. It is designed for the express purpose of toning and firming neglected muscles that cause sagging tissues.

I had a dual purpose in perfecting MultiToner. One, that it would give you the results you want; and two, it would not be just another exercise aid that ends up in the closet.

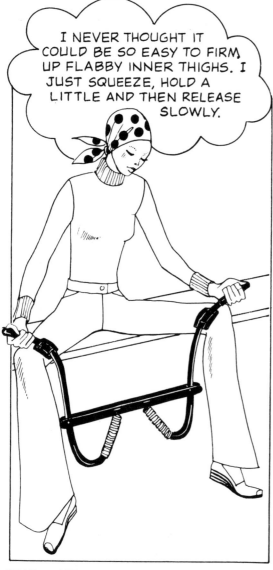

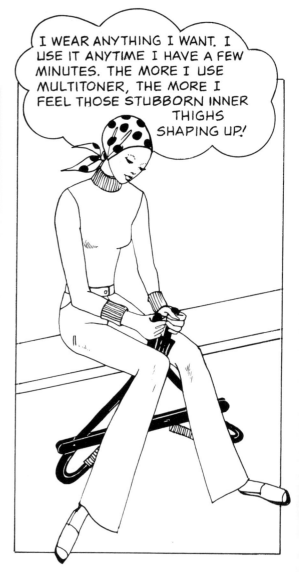

*MultiToner, 987 Lexington Avenue, New York, N.Y. 10021.

YOU AND YOUR PELVIS

"Pelvis" is the technical term that describes the center of the body. It starts at the top of the hip bone and ends at the hip joint. It covers a lot of territory, the lower stomach, lower back and hips.

The pelvis is a key area. It should be held straight, both for your beauty and your well-being. To keep it erect, think of the pelvic area as a large punch bowl, filled. And you don't want anything to spill out. A pelvis out of place can cause quite a few figure faults. Pelvic exercises not only help to correct these faults, they're easy to do and so relaxing!

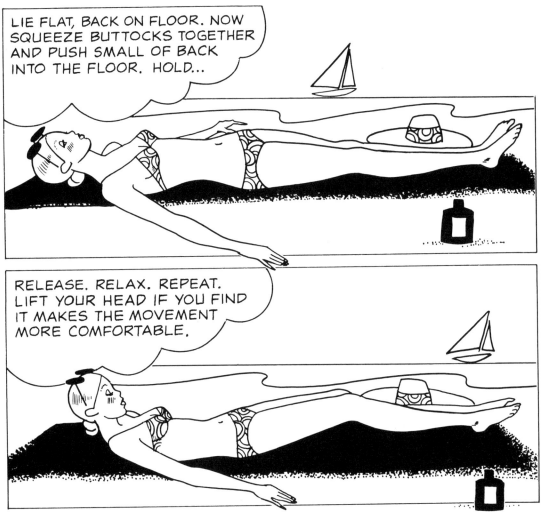

TIP: This is a great way to break the "refrigerator syndrome" when watching a TV special!

MEET YOUR PELVIS

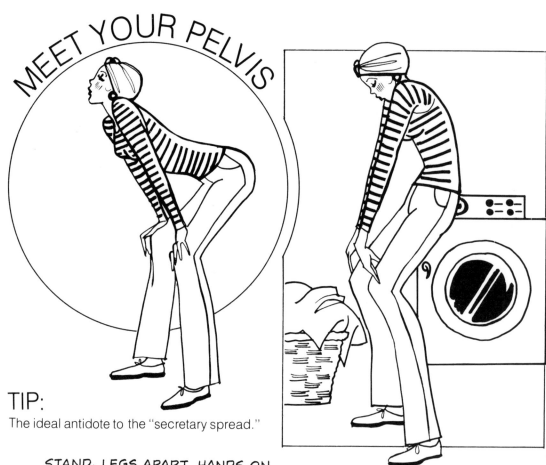

TIP:
The ideal antidote to the "secretary spread."

STAND, LEGS APART, HANDS ON
KNEES. KEEP YOUR HEAD UP. THEN
SWING ENTIRE PELVIS FORWARD IN ONE SMOOTH MOVEMENT.
TIGHTEN BUTTOCKS, INNER THIGHS AND STOMACH AS YOU MOVE
HOLD TO A COUNT OF 5, RETURN TO STARTING POSITION. REPEAT
ENTIRE MOVEMENT 5 TIMES.

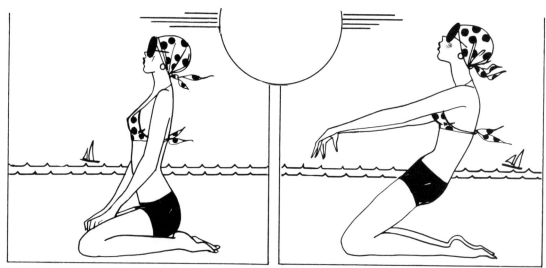

KNEEL DOWN AND SIT ON YOUR HEELS. ARCH YOUR BACK
SLIGHTLY. NOW RISE UP A LITTLE, PUSHING PELVIS FOWARD
WITH BUTTOCKS HELD TIGHT. HOLD INNER THIGHS AND
STOMACH TIGHT AT THE SAME TIME. RELEASE SLOWLY. RELAX.
REST. REPEAT.

TIP: Try it whenever something rolls under the bed, table, or sofa.

YOU AND YOUR BUTTOCKS

Alas! It seems to be a rarity—that extremely attractive feature of a woman's body—a taut, shapely behind.

On most women, it's out of shape. Flabby, flattened, flaring, falling, etc., etc., etc.

Yet it doesn't take all that much to firm and lift it up. But, you must know how. That's the real secret.

Think how we mistreat, misuse our buttocks. We sit on them to excess. We bind them in girdles, pants, skirts, hose that don't fit and squeeze them out of shape. We don't give them a chance to stay shapely with a little on-the-spot exercise . . . especially considering that the pull of gravity works against them and tends to add a bulge on the upper thigh. In other words, it's total neglect.

Give your buttocks a chance.

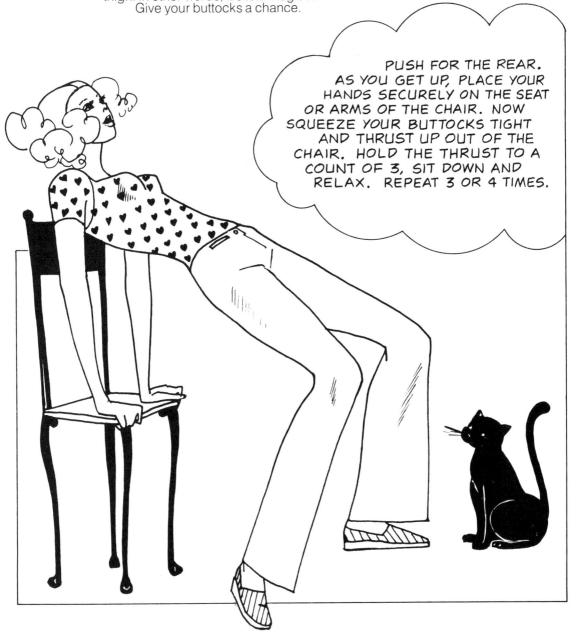

PUSH FOR THE REAR. AS YOU GET UP, PLACE YOUR HANDS SECURELY ON THE SEAT OR ARMS OF THE CHAIR. NOW SQUEEZE YOUR BUTTOCKS TIGHT AND THRUST UP OUT OF THE CHAIR. HOLD THE THRUST TO A COUNT OF 3, SIT DOWN AND RELAX. REPEAT 3 OR 4 TIMES.

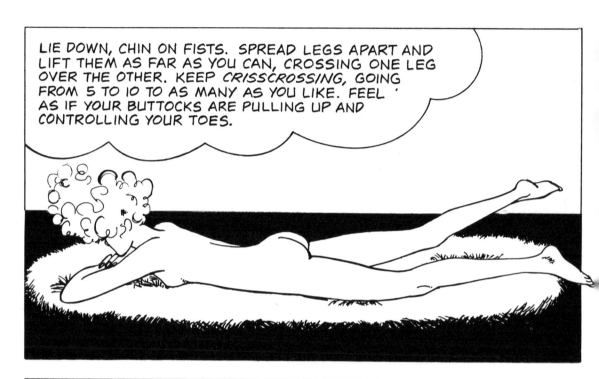

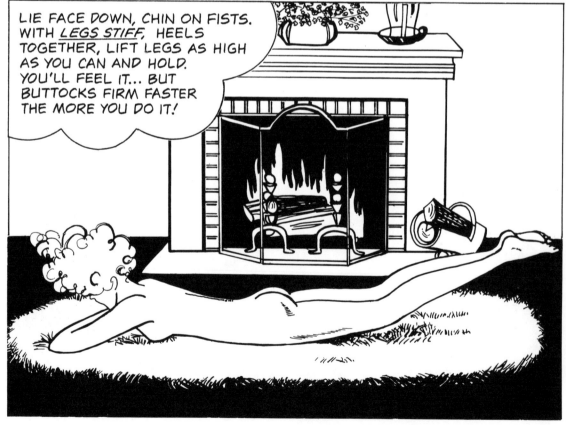

THE SUPER LIFT

Choose your support—a crib,
kitchen counter, bathroom sink,
filing cabinet—anything at least
waist-high and sturdy. With feet
about 6 inches away, lean flat
against your support. That
arches your back, helps you
tuck your buttocks in and
under. Now raise your leg out
and back. Bounce the leg up
and down about 10 times to
start. Do the other leg after
shifting your weight. You can
also make small circles with
each leg. I call this the "Super
Lift" because that's what it does
for your buttocks. Practice this
whenever you have even a few
seconds and some support. It
can make quite a difference in
your shape!

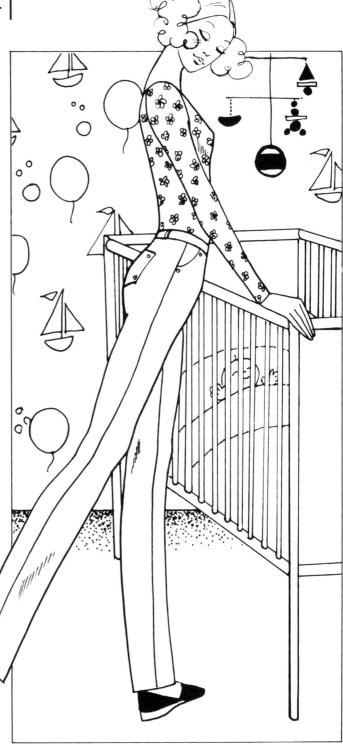

YOU AND YOUR STOMACH

Some lucky people are born with flat stomachs. But even they gamble with their luck if they "practice" bad posture. Such a common out-of-shape area, and all too often the result of sloppy habits.

Stomach exercises don't have to be the boring old sit-ups and leg-ups to show results. They do have to be the right ones to build strong stomach muscles. To accomplish this, the small of the back must be pressed flat against the floor when doing exercises lying down. Shoulders must be rounded when doing exercises sitting on the floor. Stomach muscles must be pulled in as if you were trying to raise your pubic bone. This way you are sure that the *stomach* muscles—not the back muscles—are doing the work. And you are sure of getting results.

If not properly done, stomach exercises can do more harm than good. Too much strain is put on the back muscles, which can cause lower back pains. They also don't show results. Correctly done, they will firm saggy muscles, flatten protruding pouches, help eliminate other unattractive side effects: digestive disorders and lack of energy, just to mention a few. Get going!

GET TO KNOW YOUR STOMACH MUSCLES

LYING ON THE FLOOR, THE BED OR A SLANT BOARD:
IMAGINE THAT YOUR STOMACH IS FLAT AGAINST YOUR
SPINE. PULL IT IN-IN-IN. ROUND YOUR SHOULDERS AND
HEAD, THEN LIFT AND REACH FOR YOUR KNEES. *CONTROL
THE MOTION WITH FIRM STOMACH MUSCLES.* HOLD.
SLOWLY GO BACK TO FLAT POSITION. AT FIRST, DO
THIS ABOUT 5 TIMES. WHEN YOU CAN CONTROL YOUR
STOMACH, RAISE YOURSELF HIGHER... AND HIGHER TO
KEEP THAT TUMMY FLAT!

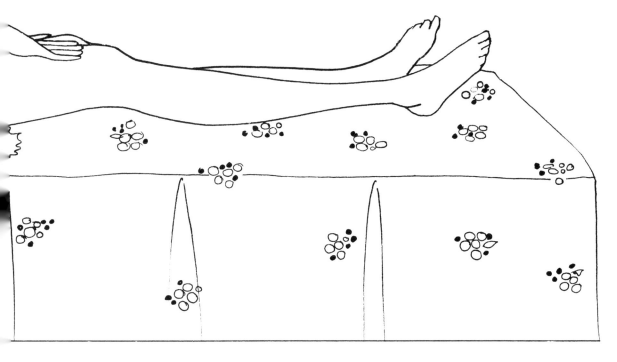

THE TUMMY FLATTENERS

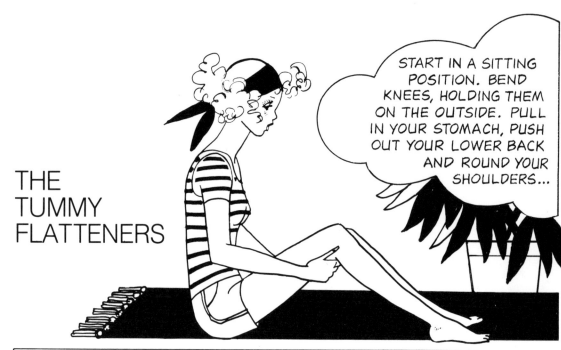

START IN A SITTING POSITION. BEND KNEES, HOLDING THEM ON THE OUTSIDE. PULL IN YOUR STOMACH, PUSH OUT YOUR LOWER BACK AND ROUND YOUR SHOULDERS...

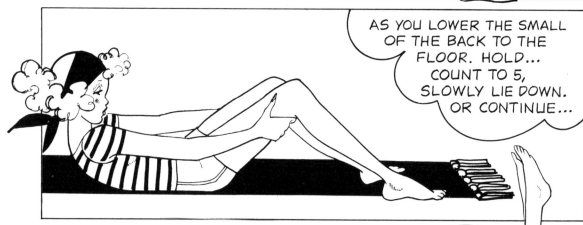

AS YOU LOWER THE SMALL OF THE BACK TO THE FLOOR. HOLD... COUNT TO 5, SLOWLY LIE DOWN. OR CONTINUE...

STOP

None of this will do you any good unless you CONCENTRATE on pulling your stomach IN. To keep up progress, build your holding time to 20 slow counts.

WITH FULL TUMMY CONTROL, SMALL OF BACK ON FLOOR, RAISE BOTH LEGS STRAIGHT UP. SPREAD APART 4 OR 5 TIMES. THEN RELAX.

TIPS for a flat stomach:

Eat slowly.
Avoid that bloated feeling.
Avoid too much bread, pasta, etc.
Skip all carbonated drinks.
Do not drink with meals.
Always sit up straight, stomach in. Don't slump.
Always pull your stomach in . . . standing, walking, bending, etc.

Here's how to get the "Flat Stomach" Habit:
Pull tummy against spine. Hold it there for a few seconds. Then slowly release. Repeat a few times in a row. Repeat daily at least for one week. The more you do it, the easier it is to keep the habit.

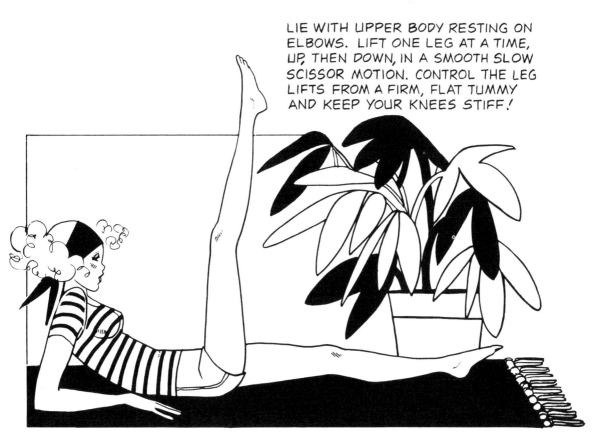

LIE WITH UPPER BODY RESTING ON ELBOWS. LIFT ONE LEG AT A TIME, UP, THEN DOWN, IN A SMOOTH SLOW SCISSOR MOTION. CONTROL THE LEG LIFTS FROM A FIRM, FLAT TUMMY AND KEEP YOUR KNEES STIFF!

YOU AND YOUR BACK

How much attention do you pay to your back—unless it hurts? Your whole body hangs from your back and slumping throws it out of whack, platform wedges strain it, a weak tummy puts it out of line. Vice versa—weak back muscles tend to make the tummy protrude.

How often do you take a rear view? Look closely to see if flab has collected around the bra or the waist? Check for protruding bones? Or do you have a back to be proud of?

P.S. Remember that unnecessary tension lands in the back. Unnecessary because proper posture prevents tension and its aches and pains. If you haven't been careful, then stretch to release tension.

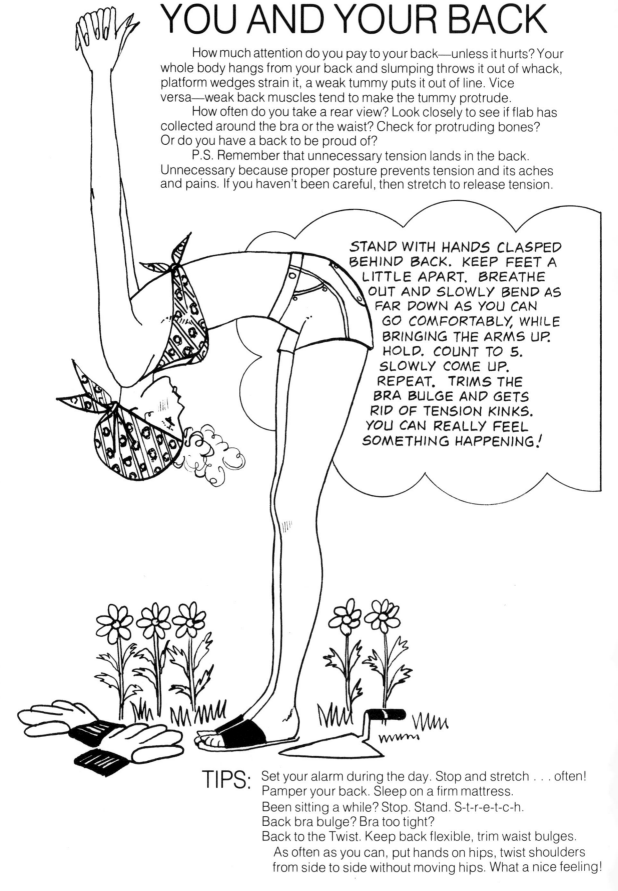

STAND WITH HANDS CLASPED BEHIND BACK. KEEP FEET A LITTLE APART. BREATHE OUT AND SLOWLY BEND AS FAR DOWN AS YOU CAN GO COMFORTABLY, WHILE BRINGING THE ARMS UP. HOLD. COUNT TO 5. SLOWLY COME UP. REPEAT. TRIMS THE BRA BULGE AND GETS RID OF TENSION KINKS. YOU CAN REALLY FEEL SOMETHING HAPPENING!

TIPS: Set your alarm during the day. Stop and stretch . . . often! Pamper your back. Sleep on a firm mattress.
Been sitting a while? Stop. Stand. S-t-r-e-t-c-h.
Back bra bulge? Bra too tight?
Back to the Twist. Keep back flexible, trim waist bulges.
As often as you can, put hands on hips, twist shoulders from side to side without moving hips. What a nice feeling!

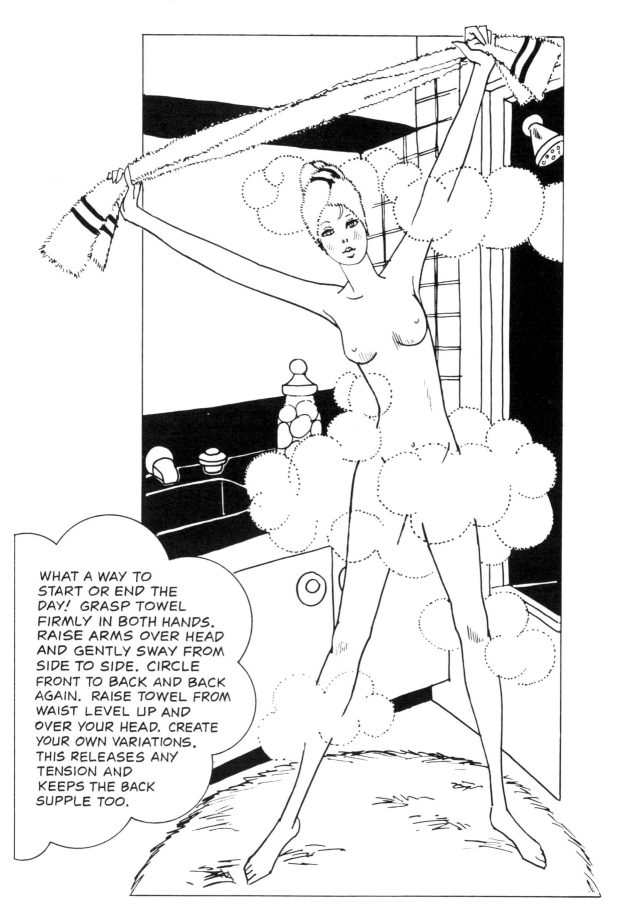

WHAT A WAY TO
START OR END THE
DAY! GRASP TOWEL
FIRMLY IN BOTH HANDS.
RAISE ARMS OVER HEAD
AND GENTLY SWAY FROM
SIDE TO SIDE. CIRCLE
FRONT TO BACK AND BACK
AGAIN. RAISE TOWEL FROM
WAIST LEVEL UP AND
OVER YOUR HEAD. CREATE
YOUR OWN VARIATIONS.
THIS RELEASES ANY
TENSION AND
KEEPS THE BACK
SUPPLE TOO.

YOU AND YOUR UPPER ARMS

Little things can give you away. Like flabby upper arms that make you look old before your time. I hate to say this but, with this particular area, prevention is the better part of wisdom. Once flab collects it is difficult to move it away. So be smart. Do some little things that can keep flab away.

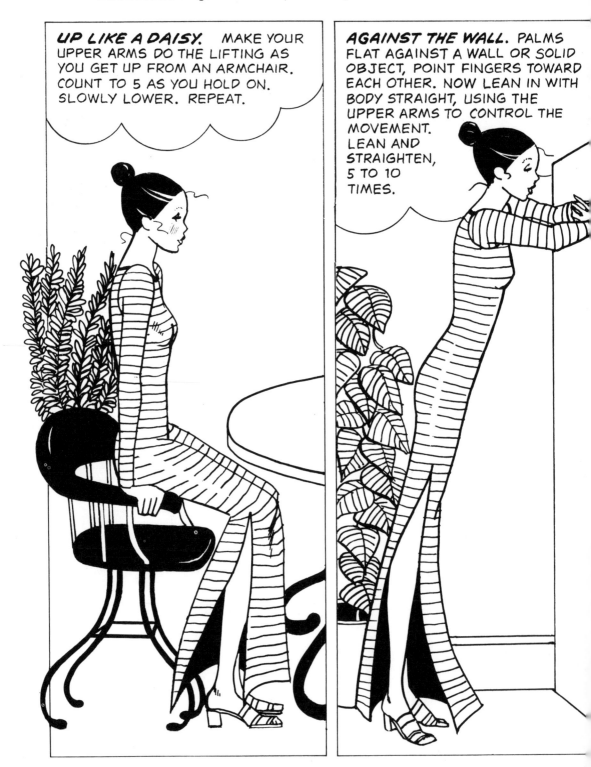

UP LIKE A DAISY. MAKE YOUR UPPER ARMS DO THE LIFTING AS YOU GET UP FROM AN ARMCHAIR. COUNT TO 5 AS YOU HOLD ON. SLOWLY LOWER. REPEAT.

AGAINST THE WALL. PALMS FLAT AGAINST A WALL OR SOLID OBJECT, POINT FINGERS TOWARD EACH OTHER. NOW LEAN IN WITH BODY STRAIGHT, USING THE UPPER ARMS TO CONTROL THE MOVEMENT. LEAN AND STRAIGHTEN, 5 TO 10 TIMES.

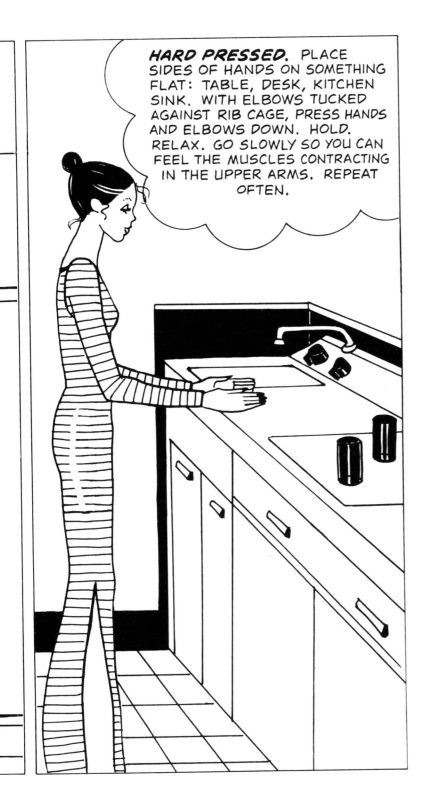

HARD PRESSED. PLACE SIDES OF HANDS ON SOMETHING FLAT: TABLE, DESK, KITCHEN SINK. WITH ELBOWS TUCKED AGAINST RIB CAGE, PRESS HANDS AND ELBOWS DOWN. HOLD. RELAX. GO SLOWLY SO YOU CAN FEEL THE MUSCLES CONTRACTING IN THE UPPER ARMS. REPEAT OFTEN.

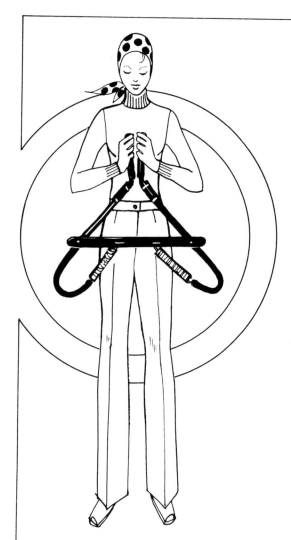

A SHORT CUT

HERE'S WHERE THE MULTITONER CAN ALSO COME TO YOUR RESCUE. IT GETS TO THOSE NEGLECTED UPPER ARMS, WORKS ON THE HARD-TO-REACH BACK AREA UP NEAR THE SHOULDER WHERE UNSIGHTLY BULGES COLLECT AROUND THE BRA.

THE ACTION OF MULTITONER GIVES MUSCLES FULL CON-TRACTION AND RELEASE. YOU SEE A NEW SMOOTHNESS, FEEL A NEW SUPPLENESS. AND THERE'S A PLUS -- YOUR BUST GETS THE BENEFIT OF BETTER SUPPORT.

TIPS: Keep up the good work all year round. Don't wait till summer when upper arms come out of hiding.
As you pass through a doorway, stretch, tensing your upper arms.
Exaggerate your movements.

YOU AND YOUR BUST

Surely you've seen all those promises for a Hollywood bustline . . . practically overnight.

Well, no exercise can change the bust you were born with. Your breasts are glands, not muscles. Which means there is nothing there to shape up or build up.

What you *can* do is strengthen the pectorals—the bust's support system. Well-toned pectorals can actually "lift" the breasts and give them that young look. Even make them *appear* bigger without a size change.

So, hurray for the A's, the B's, the C's, the D's and the "custom" size busts! Whatever your size bust, let's keep it up.

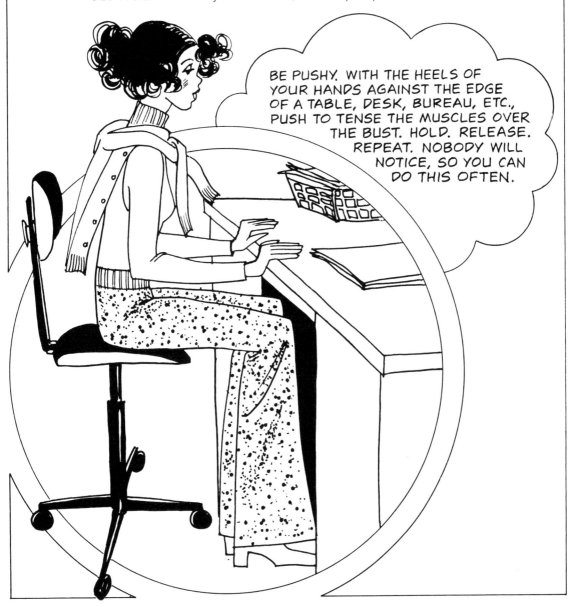

BE PUSHY. WITH THE HEELS OF YOUR HANDS AGAINST THE EDGE OF A TABLE, DESK, BUREAU, ETC., PUSH TO TENSE THE MUSCLES OVER THE BUST. HOLD. RELEASE. REPEAT. NOBODY WILL NOTICE, SO YOU CAN DO THIS OFTEN.

THE "LIBERATED" BUST...

wears a bra. Unless you happen to have *very* strong pectoral muscles or *tiny* breasts, wearing a bra—one that gives good support—is a must.

The "little nothing" bras made out of stretch fabrics are worthless, in fact detrimental. Because they offer no support, they can do more harm than good. A good supporting bra doesn't mean a harness. It can and should be attractive.

Going bra-less might be "sexy" when you're young, although there's nothing sexy about large, pendulous breasts that flop around under a shirt. Only women with small, firm breasts can afford that. Really. On a special occasion, if you want to look and feel particularly devastating, fine, you can skip wearing a bra. But not all day, not everyday.

Think what can happen to you in the long run. No support. No foundation. And your bust falls, droops, sags. In time, lets you down completely.

HERE ARE A FEW TIPS:

- You've heard it before, but I repeat . . . good posture is terribly important. Slouching and hunching do nothing for your breasts except deteriorate them a little more everyday. My suggestion: try wearing a sexy, lacy bra and maybe leave a strategic button open so it peeks through. A good way to remind yourself to straighten up.
- Never wear your bra too tight. This bad habit is responsible for the unsightly "bra bulge." You just create more lumps. My suggestion: Ask for help when you buy a new bra. A trained salesperson can guide you to the correct fit.
- Keep your shape natural. Don't adjust the straps so your bust meets your chin!
- In order for the bustline to be in good shape, the muscles of the back must also be in good shape. Here are some sports that can be particularly helpful for both bust and back: swimming, volleyball, rowing, tennis.
- The traditional palm-squeeze usually suggested to strengthen the pectorals is unfortunately limiting. Try this variation to build good all-around-the-bust support:
  Hold arms straight out at shoulder level. Cross hands one over the other rapidly about 10 times. Then open arms wide and bounce to the back a few times. Repeat 5 times.
- Do as the French do. Splash cold water on your breasts. (Bend over the sink and use a washcloth or sponge. Not as chilly as it sounds.) This helps tighten the skin and improves the overall tone by stimulating circulation locally.
- Double up. Whenever you work on the upper arms, your bust gets a nice workout too!

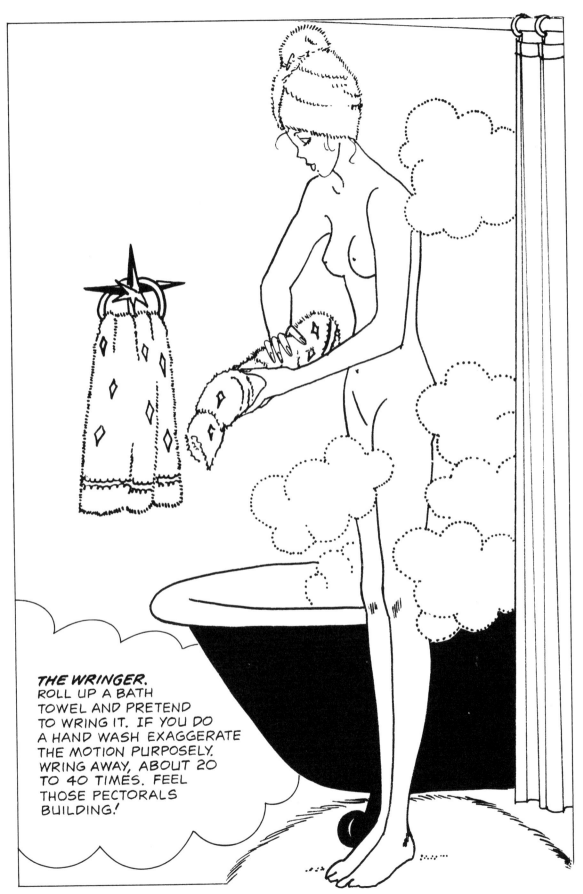

THE WRINGER.
ROLL UP A BATH
TOWEL AND PRETEND
TO WRING IT. IF YOU DO
A HAND WASH EXAGGERATE
THE MOTION PURPOSELY.
WRING AWAY, ABOUT 20
TO 40 TIMES. FEEL
THOSE PECTORALS
BUILDING!

YOU AND YOUR FACE

Just like any other part of your body, you can exercise your face. Why bother? Many lines, folds and furrows are caused by lack of muscle tone. When you add this to the downward pull of gravity, you encourage a look of premature age.

Exercise helps give the face a natural "lift!" But face exercises should not distort, stretch or add lines. They must be done sensibly and scientifically.
Prevention is the best short cut.
Don't wait until your face has become a "disaster" to start taking care of it!

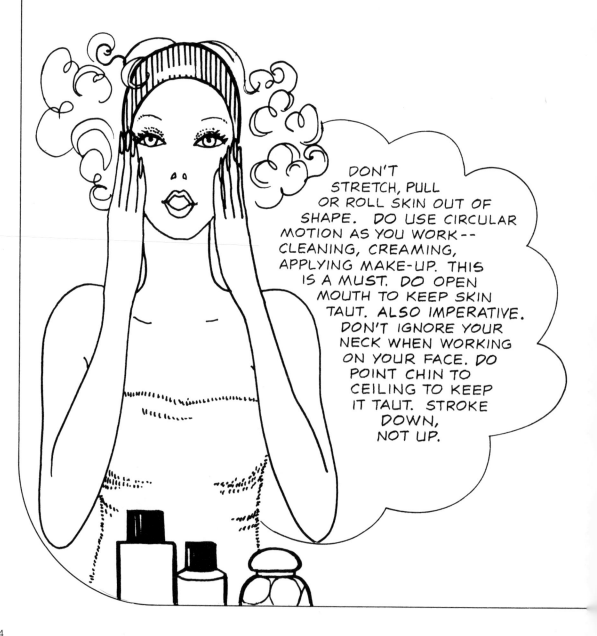

DON'T STRETCH, PULL OR ROLL SKIN OUT OF SHAPE. DO USE CIRCULAR MOTION AS YOU WORK -- CLEANING, CREAMING, APPLYING MAKE-UP. THIS IS A MUST. DO OPEN MOUTH TO KEEP SKIN TAUT. ALSO IMPERATIVE. DON'T IGNORE YOUR NECK WHEN WORKING ON YOUR FACE. DO POINT CHIN TO CEILING TO KEEP IT TAUT. STROKE DOWN, NOT UP.

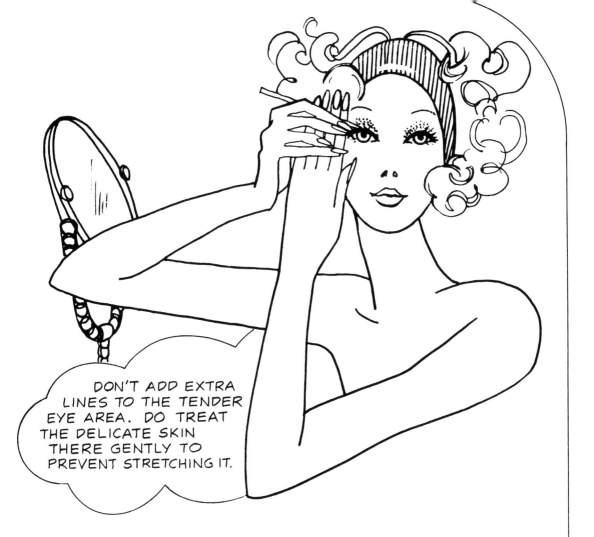

Either press skin at temples, or lift chin and look down when applying and removing eye make-up. To prevent squinting, wear sunglasses when driving, sporting, etc. And another thing: don't rub your eyes, squint or frown if you can help it.

TIPS: When brushing hair, bend over to bring fresh supply of blood to the face.

When reading or watching TV, make sure the neck is stretched, to preserve chin line.

For sleeping use no pillow, or, if you must, use one as flat as possible.

The surest way to preserve a swan-like neck is through good posture. Always think of stretching your neck up, *not just your chin,* your neck.

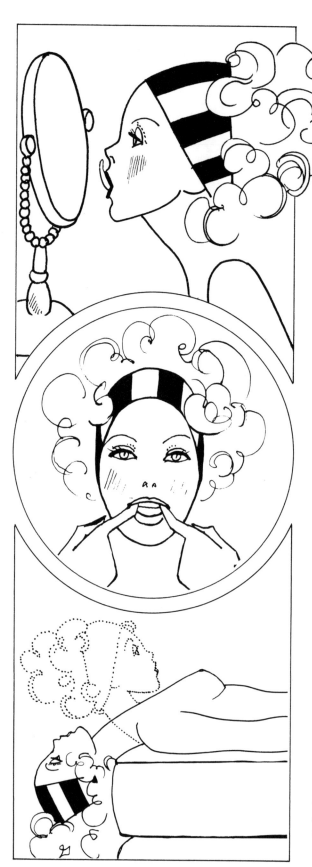

DO FACE UP

STICK OUT YOUR TONGUE TO KEEP THAT CHIN FIRM. OPEN YOUR MOUTH. TENSE YOUR JAW AND FORCE YOUR TONGUE OUT, FIRST UP, THEN DOWN. "TRY" TO TOUCH NOSE AND CHIN. KEEP THROAT MUSCLES TENSE AT LEAST 10 SECONDS.

PLUMP OUT THOSE LAUGH LINES. HOOK FIRST JOINT OF INDEX FINGERS UNDER LAUGH LINES. TRY TO CLOSE YOUR MOUTH WHILE RESISTING WITH YOUR FINGERS. TRY IT 4 OR 5 TIMES.... JUST BEFORE OR JUST AFTER BRUSHING YOUR TEETH.

STRETCH OUT THAT NECK. DROP HEAD OVER THE EDGE OF THE BED AND LET NECK S-T-R-E-T-C-H. LIFT HEAD, CHIN TO CHEST. ROLL HEAD AROUND ON NECK, SIDE TO SIDE, BACK TO FRONT, IN CIRCLES. SO RELAXING! AND A GREAT COMPLEXION REVIVER. SEE WHAT IT CAN DO BEFORE A DATE!

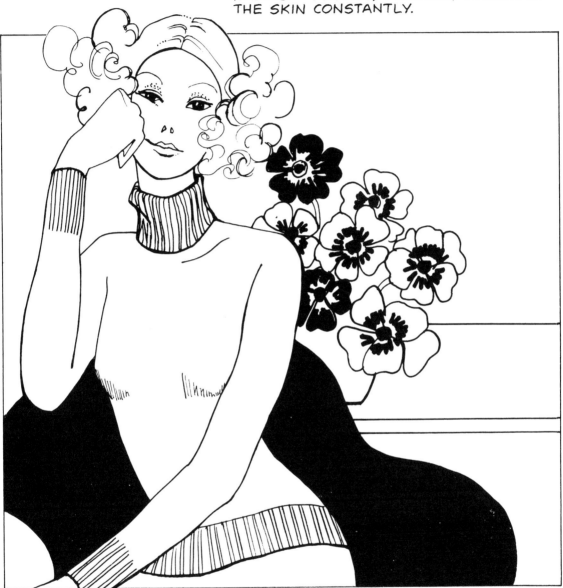

DON'T MAKE IT WORSE BY LEANING YOUR FACE ON YOUR HANDS IN WAYS THAT PULL THE SKIN. BY GIVING INTO BAD HABITS-- PICKING, PULLING, TOUCHING THE SKIN CONSTANTLY.

HELP IT ALONG

Lie on a slant board, whenever possible, to reverse that pull of gravity, encourage circulation and stimulate a fresh complexion. If you're up to it, inverted Yoga postures are splendid for the face. Avoid holding your face tense. Tension lines age you, rob you of sparkle and vitality, the glow of youth, whether you're 20 or 80.

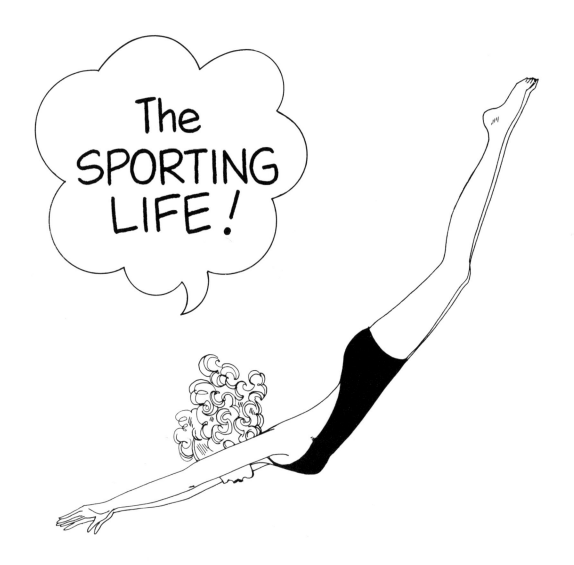

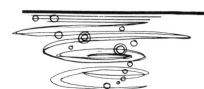

Sports are exercise—as if you didn't know! But not figure control, unless you make them work for you or unless you happen to be an all-around athlete. Here again, and I repeat, if you concentrate on your movements, get in the habit of using your movements correctly, sports can count toward a shapelier you.

All sports really exercise the whole body. Help to tone it up. But with some, you can concentrate more on the areas that need special help.

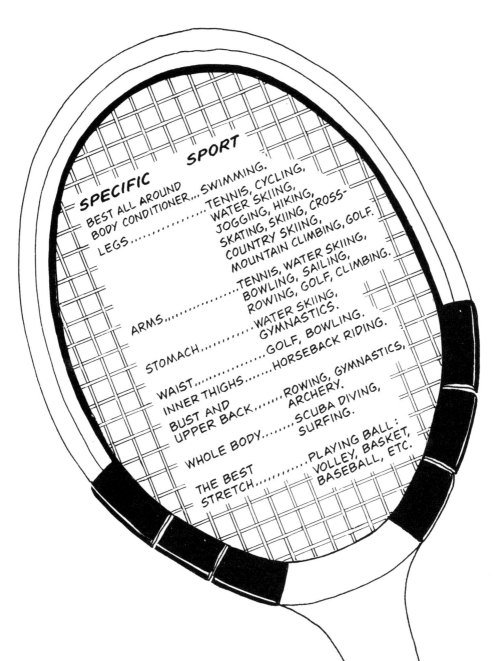

SPECIFIC SPORT

BEST ALL AROUND
BODY CONDITIONER... SWIMMING.

LEGS .... TENNIS, CYCLING,
WATER SKIING,
JOGGING, HIKING,
SKATING, SKIING, CROSS-
COUNTRY SKIING,
MOUNTAIN CLIMBING, GOLF.

ARMS .... TENNIS, WATER SKIING,
BOWLING, SAILING,
ROWING, GOLF, CLIMBING.

STOMACH .... WATER SKIING,
GYMNASTICS.

WAIST .... GOLF, BOWLING.

INNER THIGHS .... HORSEBACK RIDING.

BUST AND
UPPER BACK .... ROWING, GYMNASTICS,
ARCHERY.

WHOLE BODY .... SCUBA DIVING,
SURFING.

THE BEST
STRETCH .... PLAYING BALL :
VOLLEY, BASKET,
BASEBALL, ETC.

TIPS:

CYCLING:
Adjust pedals to the full length of your legs. This is a MUST for good cycling and the only way to give the legs a good workout.

TENNIS:
Tense inner thighs as you crouch, waiting for the ball. Pull stomach in, bend knees as you pick up the balls. Stretch as you reach for the ball.

IN GENERAL:
Tense and relax muscles as you play. Don't just go through the motions. Give it that extra bit of energy. For example,
Golf: swing the club so you trim the waist. *Walk with your head* and use your whole body.

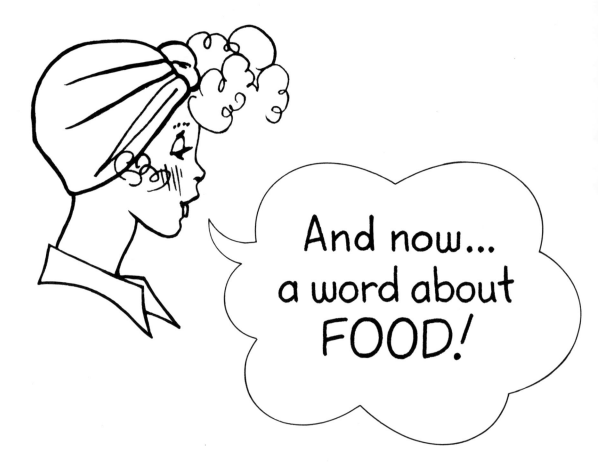

And now...
a word about
FOOD!

If you are going to make every movement count and stay in shape with daily, easy exercise, you must consider how you eat. I hear so many people complain that exercise doesn't help, only to find that they still eat big desserts, giant-size portions, high calorie snacks, "energizing" quick-lift sweets and soft drinks. Of course they don't see any results!

You are what you eat, and if you eat the wrong things you'll have the wrong shape. Buy right. Eat fresh, unprocessed foods. Fresh fruit and vegetables ... not canned varieties. Whole-grain breads, uncolored cheeses naturally processed , fresh eggs, lean meats, fish and poultry.

Cook right ... cook vegetables to crisp, not mushy texture to preserve all the vitamins and minerals. Prepare your own potatoes and rice from scratch instead of using the instant kind. Meats—broil or lightly pan sauté. Avoid rich sauces and gravies. A salad with every main meal or as a meal in itself. Fruits—fresh or dried—for dessert. And if your family insists on sweets, serve small portions. If they're homemade, at least you know what's in them!

NO-EXCUSE ENERGY FOODS

Lean meat
Poultry
Fish
Eggs
Cheese
Yogurt
Fruit, fresh & dried
Whole-grain cereal

NO-NO ENERGY FOODS

Candy bars
Soft drinks
Potato chips
Sweet, processed cereals
Processed meats
TV dinners
Gooey pastries
"Junk food" in general

THE ART OF SNACKING

Raw vegetables—carrots, beans,
    radishes, etc.
Fruits—grapes, strawberries,
    bananas, apples, pears, etc.
Yogurt
Cheese
Nuts & seeds, unprocessed

TIPS:
Eating for a Super Figure

Eat small portions.
Eat slowly.
Eat foods with variety.
Eat when you first get hungry—don't wait
    till you're starving.
And the last beautiful tip—of course
    —lots of water!

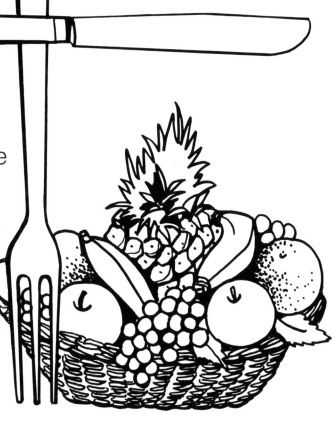

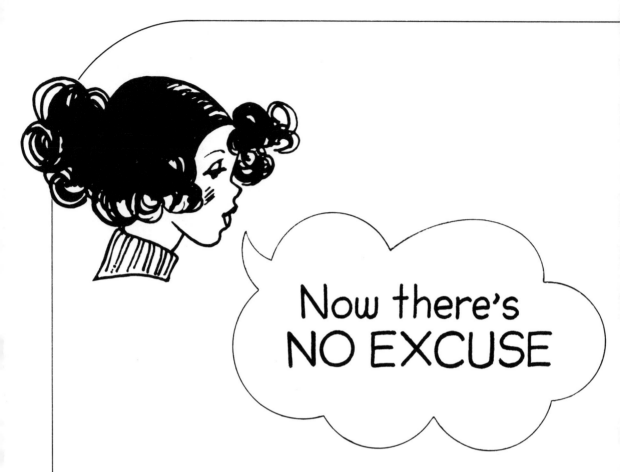

Now there's
NO EXCUSE

YOU CAN KEEP YOUR FIGURE:

AT HOME
in bed, in the bath or shower, in the kitchen, dining room, playroom; morning, noon and night; cleaning, cooking, baby sitting.

ON THE JOB
in the office, waiting on customers, in the plant, typing, packing, coding, filing, at the computer.

WAITING
for the bus, the carwash, the movies, the bank teller, the rush – hour traffic.

PLAYING
at sports, with the children, your husband, your friends, dancing, bridge, chess.

WATCHING
TV, football, baseball, the movies, the races.

By concentrating on your movements, by making every movement count towards a vibrant, alive, sensational looking you!

WHY NO EXCUSE?

I knew the plan had to be easy so women would follow it. Results would have to be quick so women would stick to it. It would have to be uncomplicated . . . no special clothes . . . no special times of day. In other words . . . any place . . . any time . . . anywhere.

My plan is for You, the modern woman. You want to enjoy every moment of your busy life without neglecting yourself. You want to feel good and look good without going out of your way. You know and I know how much better we feel after some exercise. And that means moving your body—anywhere and everywhere you happen to be.

So, these are the reasons for my *No-Excuse Exercise Guide*. The benefits are many because now you can do it. Now you have NO EXCUSE not to keep beautifully in shape!

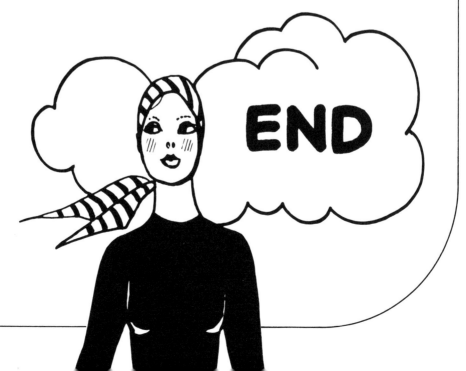